THE ATKINS DIET BIBLE

An Beginner Manual For Adopting A Low-Carbohydrate Lifestyle, With Uncomplicated Recipes And Meal Plans For Promoting Healthy Eating Habits.

CRUE GAGE

Table of Contents

Introductory

The Atkins Diet is a low-carbohydrate diet designed for weight loss and maintenance. It emphasizes the consumption of proteins and fats while significantly restricting carbohydrate intake. The diet is structured in four phases:

• **Induction Phase**: This initial phase is the most restrictive, allowing for only 20 grams of carbohydrates per day, primarily from leafy green vegetables. This phase lasts for at least two weeks and aims to kickstart weight loss by putting the body into ketosis, a state where it burns fat for energy instead of carbohydrates.

• **Balancing Phase**: During this phase, you gradually add more nuts, low-carb vegetables, and small amounts of fruit back into your diet. The goal is to find the critical carbohydrate level for losing weight, which is the number of carbs you can eat while still losing weight.

• **Pre-Maintenance Phase**: As you get closer to your goal weight, you can add more carbs back into your diet until your weight loss slows down. This helps you learn how many carbs you can eat without gaining weight.

• **Lifetime Maintenance Phase**: Once you reach your goal weight, you continue to monitor your carbohydrate intake to ensure you maintain your weight loss. This phase is about finding a balance that works for long-term maintenance.

The Atkins Diet claims to help people lose weight quickly and effectively while allowing them to eat foods that many other diets restrict, such as meats, cheeses, and fats. However, it has been controversial, with some health experts raising concerns about its high fat and protein content, potential nutrient deficiencies, and long-term sustainability.

CHAPTER ONE
Key Principles and Phases

The Atkins Diet is based on several key principles and is divided into four distinct phases. Here's a detailed breakdown:

<u>Key Principles:</u>

• **Low Carbohydrate Intake**: The diet focuses on significantly reducing carbohydrate intake to encourage the body to enter a state of ketosis, where it burns fat for energy instead of carbohydrates.

• **High Protein and Fat Consumption**: Instead of carbs, the diet promotes the consumption of proteins and fats, which help in maintaining muscle mass and satiety.

- **Ketosis**: By limiting carbs, the body enters ketosis, which is believed to enhance fat burning.

- **Gradual Carbohydrate Reintroduction**: Carbs are gradually reintroduced to the diet in a controlled manner to find a balance that allows for weight maintenance.

- **Personalization**: The diet emphasizes finding an individual balance of carbs that works for long-term weight maintenance and health.

<u>**Phases:**</u>

Induction Phase:

- **Duration**: At least two weeks, but can be extended.

- **Carb Limit**: 20 grams of net carbs per day, primarily from leafy greens and other low-carb vegetables.

- **Goal**: To initiate weight loss by putting the body into ketosis. This phase typically leads to rapid weight loss.

Balancing Phase:

- **Duration**: Until you are within 10 pounds of your target weight.
- **Carb Limit**: Gradually increase daily carb intake by 5 grams each week.
- **Foods Added**: Nuts, seeds, berries, and more low-carb vegetables.
- **Goal**: To continue weight loss while discovering your personal tolerance for carbohydrate intake.

Pre-Maintenance Phase:

- **Duration**: Until you reach your target weight.

- **Carb Limit**: Increase daily carb intake by 10 grams each week.

- **Foods Added**: More fruits, starchy vegetables, and whole grains.

- **Goal**: To slow weight loss as you approach your goal weight and determine the amount of carbs you can eat while maintaining your weight.

Lifetime Maintenance Phase:

- **Duration**: Ongoing, for life.

- **Carb Limit**: Maintain the level of carbs that allows you to keep your weight stable.

- **Goal**: To sustain your weight loss long-term and continue healthy eating habits. This phase emphasizes maintaining the lifestyle changes made during the diet.

Each phase of the Atkins Diet is designed to help individuals progressively adapt to a low-carb lifestyle, achieve weight loss goals, and maintain a healthy weight in the long term.

Benefits Of The Atkins Diet

The Atkins Diet offers several potential benefits, particularly for weight loss and metabolic health. Here are some of the key benefits:

Weight Loss:

• **Rapid Initial Weight Loss**: The induction phase often leads to quick weight loss, which can be motivating.

- **Sustained Weight Loss**: Many people experience continued weight loss over the long term by following the diet's phases and principles.

Improved Blood Sugar Control:

- **Reduced Blood Sugar Levels**: By limiting carbohydrate intake, the diet can help stabilize blood sugar levels, which is beneficial for people with type 2 diabetes or insulin resistance.

- **Improved Insulin Sensitivity**: The diet can enhance the body's sensitivity to insulin, helping manage and potentially prevent type 2 diabetes.

Enhanced Metabolic Health:

- **Improved Cholesterol Levels**: Some studies suggest that the Atkins Diet can improve cholesterol profiles, including increasing HDL (good cholesterol) and reducing triglycerides.

• **Lower Blood Pressure**: Weight loss and reduced carbohydrate intake can contribute to lower blood pressure.

Appetite Suppression:

• **Increased Satiety**: The high protein and fat content of the diet can lead to greater feelings of fullness, reducing overall calorie intake.

• **Reduced Cravings**: Many people find that cravings for sweets and high-carb foods diminish.

Potential Cognitive Benefits:

• **Improved Mental Clarity**: Some individuals report enhanced focus and mental clarity while in ketosis.

• **Potential Neuroprotective Effects**: Emerging research suggests that low-carb, high-fat diets like Atkins may have protective effects against neurological disorders.

Greater Food Variety:

• **Flexible Food Choices**: Unlike some other diets, Atkins allows for a wide range of foods, including meats, cheeses, and healthy fats, which can make it easier to adhere to.

<u>**Long-Term Sustainability**</u>:

• **Personalized Approach**: The gradual reintroduction of carbohydrates allows individuals to find their own carb tolerance, making the diet more personalized and sustainable long-term.

• **Focus on Whole Foods**: Emphasizing whole, unprocessed foods can promote overall health and well-being.

While the Atkins Diet has several potential benefits, it's important to consider individual health needs and consult with a healthcare professional before starting any new diet. Some people may experience side effects or find the diet challenging to maintain, and it's essential to ensure nutritional balance and adequacy.

Types Of Carbohydrates & How It Affect The Body

Carbohydrates are one of the three macronutrients essential for the body, along with proteins and fats. They are a primary source of energy and come in various forms, each affecting the body differently. Here's a detailed look at the types of carbohydrates and their impacts on the body:

Types of Carbohydrates:

Simple Carbohydrates (Sugars):

- **Monosaccharides**: The simplest form of carbohydrates, consisting of single sugar molecules like glucose, fructose, and galactose.

- **Disaccharides**: Composed of two monosaccharide molecules, examples include sucrose (table sugar), lactose (milk sugar), and maltose (malt sugar).

- **Sources**: Fruits, honey, table sugar, milk, and sugary processed foods.

- **Effects on the Body**: Simple sugars are rapidly digested and absorbed, leading to quick spikes in blood sugar levels, which can cause a rapid burst of energy followed by a crash. This can contribute to cravings and overeating.

Complex Carbohydrates (Starches and Fiber):

- **Polysaccharides**: Long chains of sugar molecules, including starches and fibers.

- **Starches**: Found in foods like potatoes, rice, bread, pasta, and legumes. They are broken down more slowly than simple sugars, providing a more sustained release of energy.

- **Fiber**: Found in fruits, vegetables, whole grains, and legumes. Fiber is not digested by the body and helps with digestion and maintaining healthy blood sugar levels.

- **Sources**: Whole grains, vegetables, legumes, nuts, seeds, and some fruits.

- **Effects on the Body**: Complex carbohydrates provide a more gradual and steady release of glucose into the bloodstream, helping to maintain stable energy levels and reduce hunger. Fiber aids in digestion, prevents constipation, and can help lower cholesterol levels.

How Carbohydrates Affect the Body:

Energy Production:

• **Primary Energy Source**: Carbohydrates are the body's preferred source of energy, especially for the brain and muscles during exercise. Glucose derived from carbs is used for immediate energy needs or stored as glycogen in the liver and muscles for later use.

Blood Sugar Regulation:

• **Glycemic Index**: Different carbohydrates have varying effects on blood sugar levels, measured by the glycemic index (GI). High-GI foods (simple sugars) cause rapid spikes, while low-GI foods (complex carbs) result in gradual increases.

• **Insulin Response**: The body releases insulin in response to increased blood sugar levels to help cells absorb glucose. Consistent high intake of high-GI carbs can lead to insulin resistance and increase the risk of type 2 diabetes.

Satiety and Weight Management:

• **Hunger and Fullness**: High-fiber foods increase satiety, helping to control appetite and reduce overall calorie intake. Simple sugars, however, may lead to rapid hunger returns, promoting overeating.

• **Weight Control**: Complex carbs, especially those high in fiber, support weight management by providing sustained energy and reducing overeating.

Digestive Health:

• **Gut Health**: Fiber promotes healthy digestion by adding bulk to stools and facilitating regular bowel movements. It also supports the growth of beneficial gut bacteria, contributing to overall digestive health.

• **Preventing Disorders**: A diet rich in fiber can help prevent digestive disorders like constipation, diverticulosis, and colorectal cancer.

Nutrient Supply:

• **Vitamins and Minerals**: Whole food sources of carbohydrates, such as fruits, vegetables, and whole grains, provide essential vitamins, minerals, and antioxidants that support overall health.

Considerations for Carbohydrate Intake:

• **Balanced Diet**: Emphasize whole, unprocessed carbs like vegetables, fruits, legumes, and whole grains while limiting refined and sugary foods.

• **Personalized Needs**: Carbohydrate needs can vary based on activity level, metabolic health, and individual preferences. A balanced intake tailored to personal health goals is essential.

• **Monitoring Intake**: For those following specific diets like the Atkins Diet, monitoring and adjusting carb intake is crucial to achieving desired health outcomes.

Understanding the types of carbohydrates and their effects on the body can help individuals make informed dietary choices to support overall health and well-being.

CHAPTER TWO

Carbohydrate Counting And Net Carbs

Carbohydrate Counting:

Carbohydrate counting is a method used to manage carbohydrate intake, particularly beneficial for people with diabetes or those following specific diets like Atkins. It involves tracking the number of grams of carbohydrates consumed in each meal and snack. Here's how it works:

• **Read Nutrition Labels**: Check the total carbohydrate content listed on the nutrition facts panel of food packages. This includes all types of carbs: sugars, starches, and fiber.

• **Understand Serving Sizes**: Pay attention to the serving size on the label and adjust the carb count according to the actual portion you consume.

• **Calculate Total Carbs**: Sum up the total grams of carbohydrates consumed throughout the day to stay within your target range.

• **Use Carbohydrate Lists**: For foods without labels, use carbohydrate counting books or apps that provide the carb content of various foods.

• **Meal Planning**: Plan meals and snacks to distribute carbohydrate intake evenly throughout the day, which helps in maintaining stable blood sugar levels.

<u>Net Carbs:</u>

• Net carbs are a concept used primarily in low-carb diets like the Atkins Diet. Net carbs refer to the amount of carbohydrates that are absorbed by the body and can affect blood sugar levels. To calculate net carbs, you subtract certain types of carbs that do not significantly impact blood sugar from the total carbohydrate count. These typically include dietary fiber and sugar alcohols.

• **Fiber**: Since fiber is not digested and does not raise blood sugar levels, it is subtracted from the total carbohydrate count.

• **Sugar Alcohols**: These are partially absorbed and have a lesser impact on blood sugar than regular sugars. Common sugar alcohols include erythritol, xylitol, and maltitol. Some people subtract all sugar alcohols, while others subtract only half, depending on their specific dietary guidelines.

<u>**Example:**</u>

- If a food item has:
- 20 grams of total carbohydrates
- 5 grams of fiber
- 2 grams of sugar alcohols

Then, the net carbs would be:

Net Carbs=20 g (total carbs)–5 g (fiber)–2 g (sugar alcohols)=13 g\text{Net Carbs} = 20 \, \text{g (total carbs)} - 5 \, \text{g (fiber)} - 2 \, \text{g (sugar alcohols)} = 13 \, \text{g}Net Carbs=20g (total carbs)–5g (fiber)–2g (sugar alcohols)=13g

<u>**Importance of Carbohydrate Counting and Net Carbs:**</u>

• **Blood Sugar Management**: For people with diabetes, counting carbs and understanding net carbs helps in managing blood sugar levels by ensuring consistent carbohydrate intake and preventing spikes.

• **Weight Loss and Maintenance**: Low-carb diets like Atkins use net carbs to help individuals stay within their carbohydrate limits, promoting weight loss and maintenance.

• **Dietary Planning**: Knowing how to count carbs and calculate net carbs allows for better meal planning, making it easier to adhere to dietary guidelines and achieve health goals.

By understanding carbohydrate counting and net carbs, individuals can make informed dietary choices that align with their health goals, whether it's managing diabetes, losing weight, or maintaining a low-carb lifestyle.

Phase 1: Induction Phase of the Atkins Diet

The Induction Phase is the first and most restrictive phase of the Atkins Diet. Its primary goal is to kickstart weight loss by putting the body into a state of ketosis. Here are the goals and guidelines for Phase 1:

Goals:

- **Initiate Weight Loss**: Rapidly begin shedding pounds by significantly reducing carbohydrate intake.
- **Enter Ketosis**: Transition the body from burning glucose for energy to burning fat, a metabolic state called ketosis.

- **Stabilize Blood Sugar**: Achieve more stable blood sugar levels and reduce insulin spikes.
- **Curb Cravings**: Reduce cravings for sugar and high-carb foods by limiting carbohydrate intake.

Guidelines:

Carbohydrate Limit:

• **20 Grams of Net Carbs per Day**: Limit daily intake to 20 grams of net carbs, primarily from vegetables.

Protein and Fat Intake:

• **Eat Liberally**: Consume adequate amounts of protein (meat, poultry, fish, eggs) and healthy fats (butter, olive oil, avocado).

Vegetable Consumption:

• **Non-Starchy Vegetables**: Focus on consuming 12-15 grams of net carbs from non-starchy vegetables like leafy greens, broccoli, and cauliflower.

Avoid Certain Foods:

• **High-Carb Foods**: Avoid grains, starchy vegetables, fruits (except for avocados, tomatoes, and olives in limited amounts), sugars, and most dairy products except cheese, cream, and butter.

Hydration:

• **Drink Plenty of Water**: Aim for at least eight 8-ounce glasses of water per day to stay hydrated and support metabolic processes.

Electrolyte Balance:

• **Maintain Electrolytes**: Consume enough salt, potassium, and magnesium to avoid imbalances, especially during the initial transition into ketosis.

Frequent Meals:

• **Regular Eating**: Eat three regular-sized meals or four to five smaller meals each day to keep hunger at bay and maintain energy levels.

Read Labels:

• **Check for Hidden Carbs**: Carefully read food labels to avoid hidden sugars and starches.

No Calorie Counting:

• **Focus on Carbs**: Instead of counting calories, focus on keeping carb intake within the set limit.

Supplements:

• **Consider Multivitamins**: Taking a multivitamin can help ensure you get essential nutrients during this restrictive phase.

<u>**Example Meal Plan for Phase 1:**</u>

• **Breakfast**: Scrambled eggs with spinach and cheese, cooked in butter.

• **Lunch**: Grilled chicken salad with leafy greens, cucumbers, and olive oil dressing.

• **Dinner**: Baked salmon with steamed broccoli and a side of cauliflower rice.

- **Snacks**: Hard-boiled eggs, cheese sticks, or a handful of nuts (within carb limits).

<u>Tips for Success:</u>

- **Meal Prep**: Plan and prepare meals in advance to avoid high-carb foods.

- **Stay Informed**: Educate yourself about which foods are allowed and which are not.

- **Listen to Your Body**: Pay attention to how your body responds and make adjustments if necessary.

- **Support**: Join support groups or forums to share experiences and get advice from others following the diet.

By adhering to these goals and guidelines, individuals can effectively kickstart their weight loss journey, transition into ketosis, and set the foundation for continued success in subsequent phases of the Atkins Diet.

Phase 1: Breakfast Recipes

Here are some breakfast recipes suitable for Phase 1 of the Atkins Diet, ensuring you stay within the 20 grams of net carbs limit per day and focus on protein and fat while minimizing carbohydrate intake.

1. Scrambled Eggs with Spinach and Cheese:

Ingredients:

- 3 large eggs
- 1 cup fresh spinach leaves
- 1/4 cup shredded cheddar cheese
- 1 tablespoon butter
- Salt and pepper to taste

Instructions:

- **Heat Butter**: Melt the butter in a non-stick skillet over medium heat.

- **Add Spinach**: Add the spinach and sauté until wilted, about 2 minutes.

- **Scramble Eggs**: In a bowl, whisk the eggs with a pinch of salt and pepper. Pour the eggs into the skillet with the spinach.

- **Cook Eggs**: Stir gently until the eggs are cooked to your liking.

- **Add Cheese**: Sprinkle the shredded cheese on top and let it melt. Serve immediately.

- **Net Carbs**: Approximately 3 grams

2. Avocado and Bacon Omelette:

Ingredients:

- 3 large eggs
- 1/2 avocado, diced

- 2 strips of cooked bacon, crumbled

- 1 tablespoon butter

- Salt and pepper to taste

Instructions:

- **Prepare Ingredients**: Cook the bacon until crispy, then crumble it. Dice the avocado.

- **Heat Butter**: Melt the butter in a non-stick skillet over medium heat.

- **Scramble Eggs**: In a bowl, whisk the eggs with a pinch of salt and pepper. Pour the eggs into the skillet.

- **Add Fillings**: As the eggs begin to set, add the crumbled bacon and diced avocado on one half of the omelette.

- **Fold Omelette**: Fold the omelette in half and cook until the eggs are fully set. Serve immediately.
- **Net Carbs**: Approximately 4 grams

3. Keto Pancakes:

Ingredients:

- 2 large eggs
- 2 ounces cream cheese, softened
- 1/2 teaspoon baking powder
- 1/2 teaspoon vanilla extract
- Butter for cooking

Instructions:

- **Blend Ingredients**: In a blender, combine the eggs, cream cheese, baking powder, and vanilla extract. Blend until smooth.
- **Heat Butter**: Melt butter in a non-stick skillet over medium heat.

- **Cook Pancakes**: Pour small amounts of batter into the skillet to form pancakes. Cook until bubbles form on the surface, then flip and cook until golden brown.
- **Serve**: Serve with a pat of butter or a small amount of sugar-free syrup if desired.
- **Net Carbs**: Approximately 3 grams per serving

4. Egg Muffins with Sausage and Cheese:

Ingredients:

- 6 large eggs
- 1/2 cup cooked sausage, crumbled
- 1/2 cup shredded cheddar cheese
- 1/4 cup heavy cream
- Salt and pepper to taste
- Non-stick cooking spray

Instructions:

- **Preheat Oven**: Preheat the oven to 350°F (175°C). Grease a muffin tin with non-stick cooking spray.

- **Mix Ingredients**: In a bowl, whisk the eggs with heavy cream, salt, and pepper. Stir in the cooked sausage and shredded cheese.

- **Fill Muffin Tin**: Pour the egg mixture into the muffin tin, filling each cup about 3/4 full.

- **Bake**: Bake for 20-25 minutes, or until the egg muffins are set and golden brown.

- **Serve**: Let cool slightly before removing from the tin. Serve warm.

- **Net Carbs**: Approximately 2 grams per muffin

5. Smoked Salmon and Cream Cheese Roll-Ups:

Ingredients:

- 4 ounces smoked salmon
- 2 ounces cream cheese, softened
- 1 tablespoon fresh dill, chopped
- 1 tablespoon capers, drained
- Lemon wedges for serving

Instructions:

- **Prepare Ingredients**: Spread the softened cream cheese evenly over the smoked salmon slices.
- **Add Fillings**: Sprinkle the chopped dill and capers over the cream cheese.
- **Roll-Up**: Carefully roll up the salmon slices.

- **Serve**: Serve the roll-ups with lemon wedges on the side.

- **Net Carbs**: Approximately 2 grams

These recipes are designed to provide variety and flavor while keeping carbohydrate intake low, helping you stay on track during Phase 1 of the Atkins Diet.

Phase 1: Lunch Recipes

Here are some lunch recipes suitable for Phase 1 of the Atkins Diet, focusing on low-carb, high-protein, and high-fat ingredients to keep you satisfied and help maintain ketosis.

1. Grilled Chicken Salad:

Ingredients:

- 2 boneless, skinless chicken breasts
- 4 cups mixed greens (lettuce, spinach, arugula)
- 1/2 cucumber, sliced
- 1/2 avocado, diced
- 1/4 cup cherry tomatoes, halved
- 2 tablespoons olive oil
- 1 tablespoon lemon juice
- Salt and pepper to taste

Instructions:

- **Season Chicken**: Season the chicken breasts with salt and pepper.

- **Grill Chicken**: Grill the chicken breasts over medium-high heat until fully cooked, about 6-7 minutes per side. Let rest and then slice.

- **Prepare Salad**: In a large bowl, combine mixed greens, cucumber, avocado, and cherry tomatoes.

- **Make Dressing**: In a small bowl, whisk together olive oil, lemon juice, salt, and pepper.

- **Assemble**: Top the salad with grilled chicken slices and drizzle with the dressing. Serve immediately.

- **Net Carbs**: Approximately 5 grams

2. Tuna Salad Lettuce Wraps:

Ingredients:

- 1 can (5 ounces) tuna, drained
- 2 tablespoons mayonnaise
- 1 tablespoon diced celery
- 1 tablespoon diced red onion
- 1 teaspoon Dijon mustard
- Salt and pepper to taste
- 4 large lettuce leaves (Romaine or Butter lettuce)

Instructions:

- **Make Tuna Salad**: In a bowl, combine the tuna, mayonnaise, celery, red onion, Dijon mustard, salt, and pepper. Mix well.
- **Assemble Wraps**: Spoon the tuna salad onto the center of each lettuce leaf.

- **Serve**: Fold the lettuce leaves around the filling to form wraps. Serve immediately.

- **Net Carbs**: Approximately 2 grams per wrap

3. Egg Salad Stuffed Avocados:

Ingredients:

- 4 large eggs, hard-boiled and chopped
- 2 tablespoons mayonnaise
- 1 teaspoon Dijon mustard
- 1 tablespoon chopped fresh chives
- Salt and pepper to taste
- 2 ripe avocados, halved and pitted

Instructions:

- **Make Egg Salad**: In a bowl, combine the chopped eggs,

mayonnaise, Dijon mustard, chives, salt, and pepper. Mix well.

- **Prepare Avocados**: Halve the avocados and remove the pits.
- **Stuff Avocados**: Spoon the egg salad into the avocado halves.
- **Serve**: Serve immediately.
- **Net Carbs**: Approximately 3 grams per half avocado

4. Zucchini Noodles with Pesto and Shrimp:

Ingredients:

- 2 medium zucchinis, spiralized
- 1/2 pound shrimp, peeled and deveined
- 2 tablespoons olive oil
- 1/4 cup prepared pesto (ensure it's low-carb)
- Salt and pepper to taste

Instructions:

- **Cook Shrimp**: In a large skillet, heat 1 tablespoon of olive oil over medium-high heat. Add the shrimp and cook until pink and opaque, about 2-3 minutes per side. Remove shrimp and set aside.

- **Cook Zucchini Noodles**: In the same skillet, add the remaining tablespoon of olive oil and spiralized zucchini. Sauté for 2-3 minutes until tender but still firm.

- **Add Pesto**: Add the pesto to the zucchini noodles and toss to coat evenly. Season with salt and pepper.

- **Combine**: Add the cooked shrimp back to the skillet and toss with the noodles and pesto.

- **Serve**: Serve immediately.

- **Net Carbs**: Approximately 5 grams

5. Bacon-Wrapped Asparagus with Chicken:

Ingredients:

- 2 boneless, skinless chicken breasts
- 12 asparagus spears
- 6 slices of bacon
- 1 tablespoon olive oil
- Salt and pepper to taste

Instructions:

- **Preheat Oven**: Preheat the oven to 400°F (200°C).
- **Prepare Chicken**: Season the chicken breasts with salt and pepper.
- **Wrap Asparagus**: Bundle 3 asparagus spears together and

wrap with a slice of bacon. Repeat with remaining asparagus.

- **Cook Chicken and Asparagus**: In a large oven-safe skillet, heat olive oil over medium-high heat. Add the chicken breasts and cook until browned, about 4 minutes per side. Add the bacon-wrapped asparagus to the skillet.

- **Bake**: Transfer the skillet to the preheated oven and bake for 15-20 minutes, or until the chicken is cooked through and the bacon is crispy.

- **Serve**: Serve immediately.

- **Net Carbs**: Approximately 4 grams per serving

These recipes are designed to keep you within the carbohydrate limits for Phase 1 of the Atkins Diet while providing delicious and satisfying meals.

Phase 1: Dinner Recipes

Here are some dinner recipes suitable for Phase 1 of the Atkins Diet, focusing on low-carb, high-protein, and healthy fats.

1. Baked Lemon Herb Chicken:

Ingredients:

- 4 boneless, skinless chicken thighs
- 2 tablespoons olive oil
- 2 tablespoons lemon juice
- 1 teaspoon dried oregano
- 1 teaspoon garlic powder
- Salt and pepper to taste
- Lemon slices and fresh parsley for garnish

Instructions:

- **Preheat Oven**: Preheat the oven to 375°F (190°C).

- **Marinate Chicken**: In a bowl, mix olive oil, lemon juice, oregano, garlic powder, salt, and pepper. Add chicken thighs and coat well. Let marinate for 15-30 minutes if possible.

- **Bake Chicken**: Place chicken thighs in a baking dish and pour any remaining marinade over them. Bake for 25-30 minutes or until the chicken is cooked through.

- **Serve**: Garnish with lemon slices and fresh parsley before serving.

- **Net Carbs**: Approximately 1 gram per serving

<u>**2. Stuffed Bell Peppers:**</u>

Ingredients:

- 2 large bell peppers (any color)
- 1 pound ground beef or turkey
- 1/2 cup diced tomatoes (canned, no sugar added)
- 1/4 cup onion, diced
- 1 teaspoon Italian seasoning
- 1/2 cup shredded mozzarella cheese
- Salt and pepper to taste

Instructions:

- **Preheat Oven**: Preheat the oven to 350°F (175°C).
- **Prepare Peppers**: Cut the tops off the bell peppers and remove seeds. Set aside.

- **Cook Filling**: In a skillet, brown the ground meat over medium heat. Add onion, diced tomatoes, Italian seasoning, salt, and pepper. Cook until the onion is soft and meat is fully cooked.
- **Stuff Peppers**: Fill the bell peppers with the meat mixture and place them upright in a baking dish. Top with mozzarella cheese.
- **Bake**: Bake for 25-30 minutes, or until the peppers are tender and the cheese is melted.
- **Serve**: Serve hot.
- **Net Carbs**: Approximately 4 grams per stuffed pepper

3. Zucchini Lasagna:

Ingredients:

- 2 large zucchinis, sliced thinly lengthwise
- 1 pound ground beef or Italian sausage
- 1 cup marinara sauce (low-sugar)
- 1 cup ricotta cheese
- 1 cup shredded mozzarella cheese
- 1 teaspoon dried basil
- Salt and pepper to taste

Instructions:

- **Preheat Oven**: Preheat the oven to 375°F (190°C).
- **Cook Meat**: In a skillet, brown the ground meat over medium heat. Season with salt, pepper, and basil. Drain excess fat.

- **Layer Ingredients**: In a baking dish, spread a layer of marinara sauce, followed by a layer of zucchini slices, then a layer of ricotta cheese. Add a layer of cooked meat and mozzarella. Repeat layers, finishing with mozzarella on top.

- **Bake**: Cover with foil and bake for 25 minutes. Remove the foil and bake for an additional 10-15 minutes until bubbly and golden.

- **Serve**: Let it cool slightly before serving.

- **Net Carbs**: Approximately 5 grams per serving

4. Cauliflower Fried Rice:

Ingredients:

- 1 medium head of cauliflower, riced (or pre-riced cauliflower)
- 2 tablespoons olive oil
- 1/2 cup diced carrots (optional)
- 1/2 cup peas (optional)
- 2 large eggs, beaten
- 2 tablespoons soy sauce (or tamari for gluten-free)
- 2 green onions, sliced

Instructions:

- **Rice Cauliflower**: If not using pre-riced cauliflower, pulse cauliflower florets in a food processor until they resemble rice grains.
- **Cook Veggies**: In a large skillet, heat olive oil over medium heat.

Add carrots and peas (if using) and sauté for 2-3 minutes.

- **Add Cauliflower**: Stir in the riced cauliflower and cook for another 5-7 minutes until tender.
- **Scramble Eggs**: Push the cauliflower mixture to the side of the skillet and add the beaten eggs. Scramble until cooked through, then mix with the cauliflower.
- **Add Sauce**: Stir in soy sauce and green onions. Cook for an additional 1-2 minutes and serve hot.
- **Net Carbs**: Approximately 5 grams per serving

5. Salmon with Garlic Butter and Asparagus:

Ingredients:

- 2 salmon fillets
- 1 bunch asparagus, trimmed
- 2 tablespoons butter
- 2 cloves garlic, minced
- Salt and pepper to taste
- Lemon wedges for serving

Instructions:

- **Preheat Oven**: Preheat the oven to 400°F (200°C).
- **Prepare Asparagus**: On a baking sheet, toss asparagus with 1 tablespoon of butter, salt, and pepper. Arrange asparagus on one side of the sheet.

- **Add Salmon**: Place salmon fillets on the other side of the sheet. Season with salt and pepper and top with minced garlic and remaining butter.
- **Bake**: Bake for 15-20 minutes, or until the salmon is cooked through and flakes easily with a fork.
- **Serve**: Serve hot with lemon wedges.
- **Net Carbs**: Approximately 4 grams per serving

These dinner recipes are designed to keep you within the carbohydrate limits for Phase 1 of the Atkins Diet while providing satisfying and delicious meals. Enjoy your healthy dining!

Phase 1: Snack Recipes

Here are some tasty snack recipes suitable for Phase 1 of the Atkins Diet, focusing on low-carb and high-protein options:

1. Cheese Crisps:

Ingredients:

- 1 cup shredded cheddar cheese (or any cheese of your choice)
- Optional: spices (like paprika, garlic powder, or Italian seasoning)

Instructions:

- **Preheat Oven**: Preheat your oven to 400°F (200°C).
- **Prepare Baking Sheet**: Line a baking sheet with parchment paper.

- **Form Crisps**: Place small mounds of shredded cheese (about 1 tablespoon each) on the baking sheet, leaving space between them. Sprinkle with optional spices if desired.
- **Bake**: Bake for 5-7 minutes or until the cheese is melted and bubbly. Let cool slightly until crisp.
- **Serve**: Enjoy as a crunchy snack.
- **Net Carbs**: Approximately 1 gram per serving

2. Celery Sticks with Cream Cheese:

Ingredients:

- 2-3 celery sticks
- 2 tablespoons cream cheese (plain or flavored)

Instructions:

- **Prepare Celery**: Wash and cut the celery sticks into bite-sized pieces.
- **Fill Celery**: Spread cream cheese inside the celery sticks.
- **Serve**: Enjoy as a refreshing and crunchy snack.
- **Net Carbs**: Approximately 2 grams per serving

3. Hard-Boiled Eggs:

Ingredients:

- 4 large eggs

Instructions:

- **Boil Eggs**: Place eggs in a saucepan and cover with water. Bring to a boil over medium-high heat.

- **Cook**: Once boiling, cover the pot and remove from heat. Let sit for 9-12 minutes, then transfer eggs to an ice bath for 5 minutes.

- **Peel and Serve**: Peel the eggs and enjoy plain, or sprinkle with salt and pepper.

- **Net Carbs**: Approximately 1 gram per egg

4. Pepperoni Chips:

Ingredients:

- 1 package of sliced pepperoni

Instructions:

- **Preheat Oven**: Preheat your oven to 400°F (200°C).

- **Prepare Baking Sheet**: Line a baking sheet with parchment paper.

- **Arrange Pepperoni**: Place pepperoni slices on the baking sheet in a single layer.

- **Bake**: Bake for 10-12 minutes or until crispy. Let cool slightly.

- **Serve**: Enjoy as a crunchy snack.

- **Net Carbs**: Approximately 1 gram per serving

5. Guacamole with Cucumber Slices:

Ingredients:

- 1 ripe avocado

- 1 tablespoon lime juice

- Salt and pepper to taste

- 1 small cucumber, sliced

Instructions:

- **Make Guacamole**: In a bowl, mash the avocado and mix in lime juice, salt, and pepper.

- **Serve with Cucumber**: Use cucumber slices as dippers for the guacamole.

- **Net Carbs**: Approximately 4 grams (for guacamole and cucumber slices)

These snacks are quick to prepare and perfect for keeping you satisfied between meals while adhering to the guidelines of Phase 1 of the Atkins Diet. Enjoy!

CHAPTER THREE
Phase 2: Balancing, Gradually Adding Carbs

Phase 2: Balancing and Gradually Adding Carbs

Phase 2 of the Atkins Diet, also known as the Balancing Phase, focuses on gradual carbohydrate reintroduction while monitoring your body's response. Here are the key principles and guidelines for this phase:

Goals:

• **Achieve Sustainable Weight Loss**: Continue losing weight while transitioning to a more balanced approach to carbohydrates.

• **Identify Personal Carb Threshold**: Determine how many carbohydrates you can consume while still maintaining ketosis.

• **Incorporate More Foods**: Reintroduce healthy, nutrient-dense carbohydrate sources without triggering cravings or weight gain.

Guidelines:

Increase Carbohydrate Intake:

• **Add 5-10 Net Carbs Weekly**: Start by adding 5-10 grams of net carbs each week. Focus on whole foods, such as vegetables, nuts, seeds, and berries.

Track Your Intake:

• **Use a Food Journal or App**: Keep track of your daily net carb intake, along with any weight changes or physical symptoms.

Incorporate Whole Foods:

• **Focus on Nutrient-Dense Options**: Introduce foods like leafy greens, berries, and low-carb vegetables. Avoid high-sugar and processed carbohydrates.

Monitor Ketosis:

• **Use Ketone Testing**: Consider testing for ketones using urine strips or blood meters to ensure you remain in ketosis as you add carbs.

Listen to Your Body:

• **Adjust Based on Responses**: Pay attention to how your body responds to the added carbohydrates. If weight loss stalls or cravings increase, consider reducing carb intake.

Continue Healthy Fats and Protein:

• **Maintain High Protein and Healthy Fats**: Continue to consume adequate amounts of protein and healthy fats to support satiety and energy.

Regular Physical Activity:

• **Incorporate Exercise**: Continue or increase physical activity to support weight loss and overall health.

Suggested Foods for Phase 2:

• **Low-Carb Vegetables**: Broccoli, cauliflower, spinach, zucchini, bell peppers.

• **Berries**: Raspberries, strawberries, and blackberries (in moderation).

• **Nuts and Seeds**: Almonds, walnuts, chia seeds, and flaxseeds.

• **Dairy**: Full-fat cheese, Greek yogurt (unsweetened), and heavy cream.

• **Whole Grains**: Small portions of quinoa or other low-carb grains may be introduced gradually.

Example Weekly Progression:

• **Week 1**: Add 5 grams of net carbs from vegetables.

• **Week 2**: Add 5 grams of net carbs from nuts or seeds.

• **Week 3**: Add 10 grams of net carbs from berries.

By the end of this phase, you should have a better understanding of your individual carbohydrate tolerance, allowing you to move on to the next phase of the Atkins

Diet while maintaining healthy eating habits.

Phase 2: Breakfast Recipes

Here are some delicious breakfast recipes suitable for Phase 2 of the Atkins Diet, allowing for a gradual increase in carb intake while keeping meals low-carb and nutritious.

1. Avocado and Egg Breakfast Bowl

Ingredients:

- 1 ripe avocado, halved and pitted
- 2 large eggs
- Salt and pepper to taste
- 1 tablespoon olive oil
- Optional toppings: diced tomatoes, fresh herbs, or hot sauce

Instructions:

- **Cook Eggs**: In a skillet, heat olive oil over medium heat. Crack the eggs into the skillet and cook until desired doneness (sunny-side up, scrambled, or poached).

- **Prepare Avocado**: While the eggs cook, scoop the flesh from one half of the avocado into a bowl, keeping the other half for serving.

- **Season and Serve**: Mash the avocado with salt and pepper, and place it in the bowl. Top with cooked eggs and any optional toppings. Serve with the avocado half on the side.

- **Net Carbs**: Approximately 5 grams (depending on toppings)

2. Spinach and Feta Omelette:

Ingredients:

- 3 large eggs
- 1 cup fresh spinach
- 1/4 cup crumbled feta cheese
- 1 tablespoon olive oil
- Salt and pepper to taste

Instructions:

- **Prepare Spinach**: In a skillet, heat olive oil over medium heat. Add spinach and sauté until wilted, about 2-3 minutes.
- **Whisk Eggs**: In a bowl, whisk the eggs with salt and pepper.
- **Cook Omelette**: Pour the eggs into the skillet over the spinach. Cook until the edges begin to set, then sprinkle feta cheese on one half.

Fold the omelette and cook until fully set.

- **Serve**: Slide onto a plate and serve hot.
- **Net Carbs**: Approximately 3 grams

3. Berry Smoothie:

Ingredients:

- 1/2 cup unsweetened almond milk
- 1/4 cup frozen mixed berries (strawberries, blueberries, raspberries)
- 1 tablespoon chia seeds
- 1 scoop protein powder (optional)
- Ice cubes (optional)

Instructions:

- **Blend Ingredients**: In a blender, combine almond milk, frozen berries, chia seeds, and protein powder (if using). Blend until smooth.

- **Adjust Consistency**: Add ice cubes for a thicker smoothie, if desired, and blend again.

- **Serve**: Pour into a glass and enjoy.

- **Net Carbs**: Approximately 6 grams (depending on berries used)

4. Greek Yogurt Parfait:

Ingredients:

- 1 cup unsweetened Greek yogurt

- 1/4 cup mixed berries (raspberries, strawberries, or blueberries)

- 1 tablespoon chopped nuts (almonds or walnuts)

- Optional: a sprinkle of cinnamon or a sugar-free sweetener

Instructions:

- **Layer Ingredients**: In a bowl or glass, layer Greek yogurt, berries, and chopped nuts.
- **Add Flavor**: Sprinkle with cinnamon or sweetener if desired.
- **Serve**: Enjoy as a refreshing and nutritious breakfast.
- **Net Carbs**: Approximately 7 grams (depending on berries used)

5. Vegetable Frittata:

Ingredients:

- 6 large eggs
- 1/2 cup bell peppers, diced
- 1/2 cup zucchini, diced
- 1/4 cup onion, diced
- 1/4 cup shredded cheese (cheddar or mozzarella)

- 1 tablespoon olive oil

- Salt and pepper to taste

Instructions:

- **Preheat Oven**: Preheat your oven to 350°F (175°C).

- **Sauté Vegetables**: In a skillet, heat olive oil over medium heat. Add bell peppers, zucchini, and onion; sauté until soft.

- **Whisk Eggs**: In a bowl, whisk the eggs with salt and pepper.

- **Combine and Bake**: Pour the eggs over the sautéed vegetables in the skillet. Sprinkle cheese on top and transfer to the oven. Bake for 20-25 minutes or until the eggs are set.

- **Serve**: Let cool slightly, then slice and serve.

- **Net Carbs**: Approximately 4 grams per serving

These recipes are designed to offer variety and flavor while allowing for gradual carb reintroduction in Phase 2 of the Atkins Diet. Enjoy your healthy breakfasts!

Phase 2: Lunch Recipes

Here are some delicious lunch recipes suitable for Phase 2 of the Atkins Diet, allowing for a gradual increase in carbohydrate intake while keeping meals low-carb and satisfying.

1. Chicken Salad Lettuce Wraps:

Ingredients:

- 1 cup cooked chicken, shredded or diced
- 1/4 cup mayonnaise

- 1 tablespoon Dijon mustard

- 1/4 cup diced celery

- Salt and pepper to taste

- 4 large lettuce leaves (Romaine or Butter lettuce)

Instructions:

- **Mix Chicken Salad**: In a bowl, combine the cooked chicken, mayonnaise, Dijon mustard, celery, salt, and pepper. Mix well.

- **Assemble Wraps**: Spoon the chicken salad onto each lettuce leaf.

- **Serve**: Roll the lettuce leaves around the filling and enjoy!

- **Net Carbs**: Approximately 3 grams per wrap

2. Zucchini Noodles with Pesto and Cherry Tomatoes:

Ingredients:

- 2 medium zucchinis, spiralized
- 1 cup cherry tomatoes, halved
- 1/4 cup prepared pesto (check for low-carb)
- 1 tablespoon olive oil
- Salt and pepper to taste

Instructions:

- **Sauté Zucchini**: In a skillet, heat olive oil over medium heat. Add the spiralized zucchini and sauté for 2-3 minutes until tender.
- **Add Tomatoes and Pesto**: Stir in the cherry tomatoes and pesto. Cook for an additional 2-3 minutes until heated through.

- **Serve**: Season with salt and pepper, and serve warm.
- **Net Carbs**: Approximately 5 grams per serving

3. Egg and Avocado Salad:

Ingredients:

- 4 hard-boiled eggs, chopped
- 1 ripe avocado, diced
- 1 tablespoon mayonnaise (optional)
- 1 tablespoon lime juice
- Salt and pepper to taste
- Optional: chopped cilantro or green onions

Instructions:

- **Combine Ingredients**: In a bowl, combine chopped eggs, diced avocado, mayonnaise, lime juice, salt, and pepper. Mix gently to avoid mashing the avocado too much.

- **Serve**: Enjoy on its own or with lettuce leaves as wraps.
- **Net Carbs**: Approximately 4 grams per serving

4. Stuffed Bell Peppers:

Ingredients:

- 2 large bell peppers (any color)
- 1 pound ground turkey or beef
- 1/2 cup diced tomatoes (canned, no added sugar)
- 1 teaspoon Italian seasoning
- 1/4 cup shredded cheese (optional)

Instructions:

- **Preheat Oven**: Preheat the oven to 350°F (175°C).
- **Cook Filling**: In a skillet, brown the ground turkey or beef. Add diced tomatoes and Italian seasoning, and cook until heated through.
- **Stuff Peppers**: Cut the tops off the bell peppers and remove seeds. Stuff with the meat mixture and top with cheese if desired.
- **Bake**: Place stuffed peppers in a baking dish and bake for 25-30 minutes until peppers are tender.
- **Serve**: Serve hot.
- **Net Carbs**: Approximately 5 grams per stuffed pepper

<u>**5. Shrimp and Avocado Salad:**</u>

Ingredients:

- 1 pound shrimp, peeled and deveined
- 1 ripe avocado, diced
- 1 cup mixed greens
- 1/4 cup diced cucumber
- 1 tablespoon olive oil
- 1 tablespoon lime juice
- Salt and pepper to taste

Instructions:

- **Cook Shrimp**: In a skillet, heat olive oil over medium heat. Add shrimp and cook until pink and opaque, about 2-3 minutes per side. Let cool slightly.

- **Combine Salad**: In a large bowl, combine mixed greens, avocado, cucumber, and cooked shrimp.

- **Dress Salad**: Drizzle with lime juice, and season with salt and pepper. Toss gently to combine.

- **Serve**: Enjoy immediately.

- **Net Carbs**: Approximately 6 grams per serving

These lunch recipes provide variety and nutrition while allowing for gradual carb reintroduction during Phase 2 of the Atkins Diet. Enjoy your meals!

Here are some delicious dinner recipes suitable for Phase 2 of the Atkins Diet, allowing for gradual carb reintroduction while keeping meals low-carb and nutritious.

1. Grilled Lemon Herb Chicken with Asparagus:

Ingredients:

- 4 boneless, skinless chicken breasts
- 1 bunch asparagus, trimmed
- 3 tablespoons olive oil
- 2 tablespoons lemon juice
- 1 teaspoon dried oregano
- Salt and pepper to taste

Instructions:

- **Marinate Chicken**: In a bowl, mix 2 tablespoons of olive oil, lemon juice, oregano, salt, and pepper. Add chicken breasts and marinate for at least 30 minutes.

- **Grill Chicken**: Preheat the grill to medium-high heat. Grill chicken for about 6-7 minutes on each side or until cooked through.

- **Sauté Asparagus**: In a skillet, heat remaining olive oil. Add asparagus and sauté until tender, about 5-7 minutes.

- **Serve**: Plate the chicken with asparagus on the side.

- **Net Carbs**: Approximately 4 grams per serving

2. Zucchini Lasagna:

Ingredients:

- 2 large zucchinis, sliced thinly
- 1 pound ground beef or turkey
- 1 cup marinara sauce (low-sugar)
- 1 cup ricotta cheese
- 1 cup shredded mozzarella cheese
- 1 teaspoon Italian seasoning
- Salt and pepper to taste

Instructions:

- **Preheat Oven**: Preheat the oven to 375°F (190°C).
- **Cook Meat**: In a skillet, brown the ground meat. Add marinara sauce, Italian seasoning, salt, and pepper. Simmer for 5-10 minutes.
- **Layer Ingredients**: In a baking dish, layer zucchini slices, ricotta

cheese, and meat sauce. Repeat layers, finishing with mozzarella on top.

- **Bake**: Cover with foil and bake for 25 minutes. Remove foil and bake for an additional 10-15 minutes until bubbly.

- **Serve**: Let cool slightly before slicing.

- **Net Carbs**: Approximately 5 grams per serving

3. Cauliflower Fried Rice:

Ingredients:

- 1 medium head of cauliflower, riced (or pre-riced cauliflower)
- 1/2 cup diced carrots (optional)
- 1/2 cup peas (optional)
- 2 large eggs, beaten

- 2 tablespoons soy sauce (or tamari for gluten-free)
- 1 tablespoon sesame oil
- 2 green onions, sliced

Instructions:

- **Rice Cauliflower**: If not using pre-riced cauliflower, pulse cauliflower florets in a food processor until they resemble rice grains.
- **Cook Vegetables**: In a large skillet, heat sesame oil over medium heat. Add carrots and peas (if using) and sauté for 2-3 minutes.
- **Add Cauliflower**: Stir in the riced cauliflower and cook for another 5-7 minutes until tender.
- **Scramble Eggs**: Push the cauliflower mixture to the side of

the skillet and add the beaten eggs. Scramble until cooked, then mix with the cauliflower.

- **Add Sauce**: Stir in soy sauce and green onions. Cook for an additional 1-2 minutes and serve hot.

- **Net Carbs**: Approximately 5 grams per serving

4. Stuffed Portobello Mushrooms:

Ingredients:

- 4 large portobello mushrooms
- 1 cup cooked spinach, drained
- 1/2 cup ricotta cheese
- 1/4 cup grated Parmesan cheese
- 1 teaspoon garlic powder
- Salt and pepper to taste
- Olive oil for drizzling

Instructions:

- **Preheat Oven**: Preheat the oven to 375°F (190°C).

- **Prepare Filling**: In a bowl, mix cooked spinach, ricotta, Parmesan, garlic powder, salt, and pepper.

- **Stuff Mushrooms**: Place portobello mushrooms on a baking sheet. Fill each cap with the spinach mixture. Drizzle with olive oil.

- **Bake**: Bake for 20-25 minutes until mushrooms are tender and filling is heated through.

- **Serve**: Enjoy warm as a hearty dinner.

- **Net Carbs**: Approximately 4 grams per stuffed mushroom

<u>5. Baked Salmon with Dill Sauce:</u>

Ingredients:

- 2 salmon fillets
- 2 tablespoons olive oil
- Salt and pepper to taste
- 1/4 cup Greek yogurt
- 1 tablespoon fresh dill, chopped (or 1 teaspoon dried)
- 1 tablespoon lemon juice

Instructions:

- **Preheat Oven**: Preheat the oven to 400°F (200°C).
- **Prepare Salmon**: Place salmon fillets on a baking sheet. Drizzle with olive oil and season with salt and pepper.

- **Bake Salmon**: Bake for 12-15 minutes or until salmon flakes easily with a fork.

- **Make Dill Sauce**: In a small bowl, mix Greek yogurt, dill, lemon juice, salt, and pepper.

- **Serve**: Serve salmon topped with dill sauce and your choice of low-carb vegetables.

- **Net Carbs**: Approximately 3 grams per serving

These dinner recipes offer variety and flavor while adhering to the guidelines of Phase 2 of the Atkins Diet. Enjoy your meals!

Here are some tasty snack recipes suitable for Phase 2 of the Atkins Diet, allowing for a gradual increase in carbohydrates while keeping them low-carb and satisfying.

1. Cucumber and Hummus Bites:

Ingredients:

- 1 large cucumber, sliced into rounds
- 1/2 cup hummus (choose a low-carb variety)
- Optional toppings: paprika, olives, or diced bell peppers

Instructions:

- **Slice Cucumber:** Cut the cucumber into thick slices.

- **Top with Hummus**: Spread a small dollop of hummus on each cucumber slice.

- **Add Toppings**: Sprinkle with paprika or top with olives/bell peppers if desired.

- **Serve**: Enjoy as a refreshing snack.

- **Net Carbs**: Approximately 3 grams per serving (depending on hummus)

2. Cheese and Salami Roll-Ups:

Ingredients:

- 4 slices of salami

- 4 slices of cheese (cheddar, provolone, or mozzarella)

- Optional: mustard or low-carb dip

Instructions:

- **Assemble Roll-Ups**: Place a slice of cheese on top of each salami slice.
- **Roll and Secure**: Roll them up tightly and secure with a toothpick if desired.
- **Serve**: Enjoy plain or with a side of mustard or low-carb dip.
- **Net Carbs**: Approximately 1-2 grams per serving

3. Deviled Eggs:

Ingredients:

- 4 hard-boiled eggs
- 2 tablespoons mayonnaise
- 1 teaspoon mustard
- Salt and pepper to taste

- Optional: paprika or chives for garnish

Instructions:

- **Prepare Eggs**: Cut hard-boiled eggs in half lengthwise and scoop out the yolks into a bowl.
- **Mix Filling**: Mash the yolks and mix with mayonnaise, mustard, salt, and pepper until smooth.
- **Fill Egg Whites**: Spoon or pipe the yolk mixture back into the egg white halves.
- **Garnish**: Sprinkle with paprika or chopped chives if desired.
- **Serve**: Enjoy chilled.
- **Net Carbs**: Approximately 1 gram per egg half

4. Almond Butter and Celery Sticks:

Ingredients:

- 2-3 celery sticks
- 2 tablespoons almond butter (unsweetened)

Instructions:

- **Prepare Celery**: Wash and cut celery sticks into manageable pieces.
- **Spread Almond Butter**: Fill the celery sticks with almond butter.
- **Serve**: Enjoy as a crunchy and satisfying snack.
- **Net Carbs**: Approximately 4 grams per serving (depending on almond butter)
- 5. **Hard-Boiled Eggs with Avocado**

Ingredients:

- 2 hard-boiled eggs, peeled and halved
- 1/2 ripe avocado, diced
- Salt and pepper to taste
- Optional: lime juice or hot sauce

Instructions:

- **Prepare Eggs**: Halve the hard-boiled eggs and place them on a plate.
- **Top with Avocado**: Sprinkle diced avocado over the egg halves.
- **Season**: Add salt, pepper, and a squeeze of lime juice or hot sauce if desired.
- **Serve**: Enjoy as a protein-packed snack.
- **Net Carbs**: Approximately 3 grams per serving

These snack recipes provide a range of flavors and textures while adhering to the guidelines of Phase 2 of the Atkins Diet. Enjoy your healthy snacks!

CHAPTER FOUR
Phase 3: Pre-Maintenance, Fine-Tuning Your Diet

Phase 3: Pre-Maintenance – Fine-Tuning Your Diet

Phase 3 of the Atkins Diet, known as Pre-Maintenance, focuses on fine-tuning your carbohydrate intake as you approach your goal weight. The aim is to find a sustainable level of carbohydrate consumption that allows you to maintain your weight loss without reverting to old eating habits.

Goals:

- **Reach Target Weight**: Continue adjusting your carbohydrate intake to achieve your ideal weight.

- **Identify Personal Carb Threshold**: Discover the amount of carbs you can consume while still maintaining your weight.
- **Incorporate More Variety**: Gradually introduce a wider range of foods and carbohydrates.

Guidelines:

Increase Carbohydrates Gradually:

• **Add 10-15 Net Carbs Weekly**: Increase your net carb intake by 10-15 grams each week. Focus on whole foods like fruits, whole grains, and starchy vegetables.

Monitor Weight and Body Composition:

• **Track Changes**: Keep a close eye on your weight and body measurements. If weight gain occurs, consider reducing your carb intake slightly.

Prioritize Nutrient-Dense Foods:

• **Choose Whole Foods:** Focus on foods rich in nutrients, such as vegetables, fruits, lean proteins, and healthy fats. Minimize processed foods and added sugars.

Stay Hydrated:

• **Drink Plenty of Water:** Continue to drink water and consider electrolyte balance, especially as your carb intake increases.

Experiment with Carbs:

• **Introduce New Foods:** Gradually add foods like berries, legumes, whole grains (such as quinoa or brown rice), and starchy vegetables (like sweet potatoes) to see how your body responds.

Listen to Your Body:

• **Adjust Accordingly**: Pay attention to how increased carbs affect your cravings, energy levels, and weight. Make adjustments as needed.

Plan for Maintenance:

• **Develop a Sustainable Eating Plan**: Start planning how you will maintain your weight once you reach your goal, focusing on balance and moderation.

<u>Suggested Foods for Phase 3:</u>

- **Fruits**: Berries (strawberries, blueberries, raspberries), melons, and cherries (in moderation).

- **Whole Grains**: Small portions of quinoa, brown rice, or whole-grain bread.

- **Starchy Vegetables**: Sweet potatoes, butternut squash, or peas (in moderation).

- **Legumes**: Beans and lentils (in moderation).

- **Healthy Fats**: Nuts, seeds, avocados, and olive oil.

By the end of Phase 3, you should have a clearer understanding of your personal carbohydrate tolerance, which will help you transition into Phase 4: Maintenance, where you'll focus on sustaining your weight loss with a balanced approach to eating.

Phase 3: Breakfast Recipes

Here are some delicious breakfast recipes suitable for Phase 3 of the Atkins Diet, allowing for a gradual increase in carbohydrates while keeping meals satisfying and nutritious.

1. Berry Smoothie Bowl:

Ingredients:

- 1/2 cup unsweetened almond milk
- 1/2 cup frozen mixed berries (strawberries, blueberries, raspberries)
- 1 tablespoon chia seeds
- Toppings: sliced almonds, fresh berries, unsweetened coconut flakes

Instructions:

- **Blend Ingredients**: In a blender, combine almond milk, frozen berries, and chia seeds. Blend until smooth.
- **Serve**: Pour into a bowl and top with sliced almonds, fresh berries, and coconut flakes.
- **Net Carbs**: Approximately 8 grams (depending on toppings)

2. Spinach and Feta Egg Muffins:

Ingredients:

- 6 large eggs
- 1 cup fresh spinach, chopped
- 1/2 cup crumbled feta cheese
- Salt and pepper to taste
- Optional: diced tomatoes or bell peppers

Instructions:

- **Preheat Oven**: Preheat the oven to 350°F (175°C).

- **Mix Ingredients**: In a bowl, whisk eggs with salt and pepper. Stir in spinach, feta, and any optional ingredients.

- **Fill Muffin Tin**: Pour the mixture into a greased muffin tin, filling each cup about 3/4 full.

- **Bake**: Bake for 20-25 minutes or until the egg is set. Allow to cool slightly before removing from the tin.

- **Net Carbs**: Approximately 2-3 grams per muffin

3. Avocado Toast on Whole Grain Bread:

Ingredients:

- 1 slice whole grain bread (low-carb variety)
- 1/2 ripe avocado
- Salt and pepper to taste
- Optional toppings: sliced radishes, cherry tomatoes, or an egg

Instructions:

- **Toast Bread**: Toast the slice of whole grain bread until golden.
- **Prepare Avocado**: Mash the avocado in a bowl and season with salt and pepper.
- **Assemble**: Spread the mashed avocado onto the toasted bread. Add optional toppings if desired.

- **Serve**: Enjoy as a satisfying breakfast.
- **Net Carbs**: Approximately 10-12 grams (depending on bread and toppings)

4. Greek Yogurt with Nuts and Seeds:

Ingredients:

- 1 cup unsweetened Greek yogurt
- 2 tablespoons mixed nuts (almonds, walnuts, pecans)
- 1 tablespoon chia seeds or flaxseeds
- Optional: a small drizzle of honey or a sprinkle of cinnamon

Instructions:

- **Combine Ingredients**: In a bowl, combine Greek yogurt, nuts, and seeds.

- **Add Flavor**: Drizzle with honey or sprinkle with cinnamon if desired.
- **Serve**: Enjoy as a protein-rich breakfast.
- **Net Carbs**: Approximately 6-8 grams (depending on honey)

5. Vegetable Omelette:

Ingredients:

- 3 large eggs
- 1/4 cup bell peppers, diced
- 1/4 cup mushrooms, sliced
- 1/4 cup onions, diced
- 1/4 cup shredded cheese (optional)
- Salt and pepper to taste
- Olive oil or butter for cooking

Instructions:

- **Sauté Vegetables**: In a skillet, heat olive oil or butter over medium heat. Add bell peppers, mushrooms, and onions; sauté until soft.

- **Whisk Eggs**: In a bowl, whisk the eggs with salt and pepper.

- **Cook Omelette**: Pour the eggs over the sautéed vegetables. Cook until the edges start to set, then sprinkle cheese on top if using. Fold the omelette and cook until fully set.

- **Serve**: Slide onto a plate and enjoy.

- **Net Carbs**: Approximately 3-4 grams per omelette

These breakfast recipes provide a variety of flavors and textures while allowing for a gradual increase in carbohydrate intake during Phase 3 of the Atkins Diet. Enjoy!

Phase 3: Lunch Recipes

Here are some delicious lunch recipes suitable for Phase 3 of the Atkins Diet, allowing for a gradual increase in carbohydrates while keeping meals satisfying and nutritious.

1. Quinoa Salad with Chickpeas and Veggies:

Ingredients:

- 1 cup cooked quinoa
- 1/2 cup canned chickpeas, rinsed and drained
- 1/4 cup diced cucumber
- 1/4 cup cherry tomatoes, halved
- 1/4 cup bell peppers, diced
- 2 tablespoons olive oil

- 1 tablespoon lemon juice

- Salt and pepper to taste

- Fresh herbs (parsley or cilantro), optional

Instructions:

- **Combine Ingredients**: In a large bowl, mix quinoa, chickpeas, cucumber, cherry tomatoes, and bell peppers.

- **Dress Salad**: In a small bowl, whisk together olive oil, lemon juice, salt, and pepper. Pour over the salad and toss to combine.

- **Serve**: Garnish with fresh herbs if desired, and enjoy.

- **Net Carbs**: Approximately 12 grams per serving

2. Turkey and Avocado Lettuce Wraps:

Ingredients:

- 6 slices of turkey breast (deli meat)
- 1 ripe avocado, sliced
- 1/2 cup shredded carrots
- Large lettuce leaves (Romaine or Butter lettuce)
- Optional: mustard or mayo

Instructions:

- **Assemble Wraps**: Lay out a lettuce leaf and layer turkey slices, avocado, and shredded carrots.
- **Add Condiments**: Spread mustard or mayo if desired.
- **Wrap and Serve**: Roll up the lettuce leaf around the filling and enjoy as a fresh, low-carb lunch.

- **Net Carbs**: Approximately 4 grams per wrap

3. Cauliflower and Cheese Bake:

Ingredients:

- 2 cups cauliflower florets
- 1 cup shredded cheddar cheese
- 1/2 cup heavy cream
- 1/4 teaspoon garlic powder
- Salt and pepper to taste
- Optional: grated Parmesan cheese for topping

Instructions:

- **Preheat Oven**: Preheat the oven to 375°F (190°C).
- **Cook Cauliflower**: Steam or boil cauliflower florets until just tender. Drain well.

- **Combine Ingredients**: In a mixing bowl, combine heavy cream, garlic powder, salt, and pepper. Stir in half of the cheddar cheese and cooked cauliflower.

- **Bake**: Transfer to a baking dish, sprinkle with remaining cheddar and Parmesan, if using. Bake for 20-25 minutes or until bubbly and golden.

- **Serve**: Enjoy warm.

- **Net Carbs**: Approximately 6 grams per serving

4. Zucchini Noodle Stir-Fry:

Ingredients:

- 2 medium zucchinis, spiralized

- 1 cup mixed bell peppers, sliced

- 1 cup cooked chicken or shrimp

- 2 tablespoons soy sauce (or tamari for gluten-free)
- 1 tablespoon sesame oil
- 1 tablespoon sesame seeds (optional)
- Green onions for garnish

Instructions:

- **Sauté Veggies**: In a large skillet, heat sesame oil over medium heat. Add bell peppers and sauté until tender.
- **Add Zoodles**: Stir in zucchini noodles and cook for 2-3 minutes until just tender.
- **Add Protein and Sauce**: Add cooked chicken or shrimp and soy sauce. Stir well and heat through.
- **Serve**: Garnish with sesame seeds and green onions, then enjoy.

- **Net Carbs**: Approximately 7 grams per serving

5. Egg Salad with Pickles:

Ingredients:

- 4 hard-boiled eggs, chopped
- 2 tablespoons mayonnaise
- 1 tablespoon Dijon mustard
- 1/4 cup dill pickles, chopped
- Salt and pepper to taste
- Optional: lettuce leaves for serving

Instructions:

- **Mix Salad**: In a bowl, combine chopped eggs, mayonnaise, mustard, dill pickles, salt, and pepper. Mix well.
- **Serve**: Enjoy on its own or on lettuce leaves as a refreshing lunch.

- **Net Carbs**: Approximately 2 grams per serving

These lunch recipes offer variety and flavor while allowing for a gradual increase in carbohydrate intake during Phase 3 of the Atkins Diet. Enjoy!

Phase 3: Dinner Recipes

Here are some tasty dinner recipes suitable for Phase 3 of the Atkins Diet, allowing for a gradual increase in carbohydrates while keeping meals satisfying and nutritious.

1. Grilled Lemon Herb Chicken with Roasted Vegetables:

Ingredients:

- 4 boneless, skinless chicken breasts
- 1/4 cup olive oil

- 2 tablespoons lemon juice

- 2 teaspoons dried oregano

- Salt and pepper to taste

- 2 cups mixed vegetables (zucchini, bell peppers, and carrots)

Instructions:

- **Marinate Chicken**: In a bowl, mix olive oil, lemon juice, oregano, salt, and pepper. Marinate chicken for at least 30 minutes.

- **Preheat Grill**: Preheat the grill to medium-high heat. Grill chicken for 6-7 minutes per side or until cooked through.

- **Roast Vegetables**: Toss mixed vegetables in olive oil, salt, and pepper. Roast in the oven at 400°F (200°C) for 20-25 minutes until tender.

- **Serve**: Plate the grilled chicken with roasted vegetables on the side.
- **Net Carbs**: Approximately 8 grams per serving (depending on vegetables)

2. Stuffed Bell Peppers with Ground Turkey:

Ingredients:

- 4 large bell peppers (any color)
- 1 pound ground turkey
- 1 cup diced tomatoes (canned, no added sugar)
- 1/2 cup cooked quinoa (optional)
- 1 teaspoon Italian seasoning
- Salt and pepper to taste
- 1/4 cup shredded cheese (optional)

Instructions:

- **Preheat Oven**: Preheat the oven to 375°F (190°C).
- **Cook Filling**: In a skillet, brown the ground turkey. Add diced tomatoes, quinoa (if using), Italian seasoning, salt, and pepper. Cook for 5-10 minutes.
- **Stuff Peppers**: Cut the tops off the bell peppers and remove seeds. Fill each pepper with the turkey mixture. Top with cheese if desired.
- **Bake**: Place stuffed peppers in a baking dish and bake for 25-30 minutes until peppers are tender.
- **Serve**: Enjoy hot.
- **Net Carbs**: Approximately 9 grams per stuffed pepper (depending on quinoa)

3. Baked Salmon with Garlic and Dill:

Ingredients:

- 2 salmon fillets
- 2 tablespoons olive oil
- 2 cloves garlic, minced
- 1 tablespoon fresh dill (or 1 teaspoon dried)
- Salt and pepper to taste
- Lemon wedges for serving

Instructions:

- **Preheat Oven**: Preheat the oven to 400°F (200°C).
- **Prepare Salmon**: Place salmon fillets on a baking sheet. Drizzle with olive oil and sprinkle with garlic, dill, salt, and pepper.

- **Bake**: Bake for 12-15 minutes or until salmon flakes easily with a fork.

- **Serve**: Serve with lemon wedges and a side of steamed vegetables.

- **Net Carbs**: Approximately 3 grams per serving

4. Zucchini Lasagna:

Ingredients:

- 2 large zucchinis, sliced thinly

- 1 pound ground beef or turkey

- 1 cup marinara sauce (low-sugar)

- 1 cup ricotta cheese

- 1 cup shredded mozzarella cheese

- 1 teaspoon Italian seasoning

- Salt and pepper to taste

Instructions:

- **Preheat Oven**: Preheat the oven to 375°F (190°C).

- **Cook Meat**: In a skillet, brown the ground meat. Add marinara sauce, Italian seasoning, salt, and pepper. Simmer for 5-10 minutes.

- **Layer Ingredients**: In a baking dish, layer zucchini slices, ricotta cheese, and meat sauce. Repeat layers, finishing with mozzarella on top.

- **Bake**: Cover with foil and bake for 25 minutes. Remove foil and bake for an additional 10-15 minutes until bubbly.

- **Serve**: Let cool slightly before slicing.

- **Net Carbs**: Approximately 7 grams per serving

5. Cauliflower Rice Stir-Fry:

Ingredients:

- 1 medium head cauliflower, riced (or pre-riced cauliflower)
- 1 cup mixed vegetables (peas, bell peppers, carrots)
- 2 large eggs, beaten
- 2 tablespoons soy sauce (or tamari for gluten-free)
- 1 tablespoon sesame oil
- Green onions for garnish

Instructions:

- **Rice Cauliflower**: If not using pre-riced cauliflower, pulse cauliflower florets in a food processor until they resemble rice grains.
- **Sauté Vegetables**: In a large skillet, heat sesame oil over

medium heat. Add mixed vegetables and sauté for 2-3 minutes.

- **Add Cauliflower**: Stir in riced cauliflower and cook for another 5-7 minutes until tender.

- **Scramble Eggs**: Push the cauliflower mixture to the side of the skillet and add the beaten eggs. Scramble until cooked, then mix everything together.

- **Add Sauce**: Stir in soy sauce and garnish with green onions before serving.

- **Net Carbs**: Approximately 5 grams per serving

These dinner recipes offer variety and flavor while allowing for a gradual increase in carbohydrate intake during Phase 3 of the Atkins Diet. Enjoy!

<h1>Phase 3: Snacks Recipes</h1>

Here are some delicious snack recipes suitable for Phase 3 of the Atkins Diet, allowing for a gradual increase in carbohydrates while keeping snacks satisfying and nutritious.

1. Apple Slices with Almond Butter:

Ingredients:

- 1 medium apple, sliced
- 2 tablespoons almond butter (unsweetened)

Instructions:

- **Slice Apple**: Core and slice the apple into wedges.
- **Serve**: Dip apple slices into almond butter for a crunchy, sweet snack.

- **Net Carbs**: Approximately 15 grams (depends on apple type)

2. Greek Yogurt Parfait:

Ingredients:

- 1 cup unsweetened Greek yogurt
- 1/4 cup mixed berries (strawberries, blueberries, raspberries)
- 1 tablespoon chia seeds
- Optional: a drizzle of honey or a sprinkle of cinnamon

Instructions:

- **Layer Ingredients**: In a glass or bowl, layer Greek yogurt, mixed berries, and chia seeds.
- **Add Sweetener**: Drizzle with honey or sprinkle with cinnamon if desired.

- **Serve**: Enjoy as a refreshing, protein-rich snack.
- **Net Carbs**: Approximately 10 grams (depends on honey and berries)

3. Cheese and Veggie Platter:

Ingredients:

- 1 cup assorted cheese (cheddar, mozzarella, or gouda)
- 1 cup raw vegetables (carrot sticks, cucumber slices, bell pepper strips)
- Optional: hummus or guacamole for dipping

Instructions:

- **Prepare Platter**: Arrange cheese cubes and raw vegetables on a plate.

- **Serve**: Add a small bowl of hummus or guacamole for dipping if desired.
- **Net Carbs**: Approximately 6-8 grams per serving (depends on veggies and dip)

4. Hard-Boiled Eggs with Sriracha:

Ingredients:

- 2 hard-boiled eggs, peeled
- Sriracha sauce to taste
- Salt and pepper to taste

Instructions:

- **Prepare Eggs**: Slice hard-boiled eggs in half.
- **Season**: Sprinkle with salt and pepper, and drizzle with Sriracha.
- **Serve**: Enjoy as a protein-packed snack.

- **Net Carbs**: Approximately 1 gram per egg half

5. Roasted Chickpeas:

Ingredients:

- 1 can (15 oz) chickpeas, rinsed and drained
- 1 tablespoon olive oil
- 1 teaspoon paprika
- Salt and pepper to taste

Instructions:

- **Preheat Oven**: Preheat the oven to 400°F (200°C).
- **Prepare Chickpeas**: Toss chickpeas with olive oil, paprika, salt, and pepper.
- **Roast**: Spread on a baking sheet in a single layer and roast for 20-25

minutes, stirring halfway through, until crispy.

- **Serve**: Allow to cool slightly before snacking.
- **Net Carbs**: Approximately 12 grams per serving (for 1/4 cup)

These snack recipes provide a range of flavors and textures while allowing for a gradual increase in carbohydrate intake during Phase 3 of the Atkins Diet. Enjoy!

CHAPTER FIVE
Phase 4: Breakfast Recipes

Here are some delicious breakfast recipes suitable for Phase 4 of the Atkins Diet, focusing on balance and variety to help maintain your weight loss.

1. Veggie Omelette with Cheese

Ingredients:

- 3 large eggs
- 1/4 cup bell peppers, diced
- 1/4 cup spinach, chopped
- 1/4 cup shredded cheese (cheddar or mozzarella)
- Salt and pepper to taste
- Olive oil or butter for cooking

Instructions:

- **Sauté Veggies**: In a skillet, heat olive oil or butter over medium heat. Add bell peppers and spinach; cook until softened.
- **Whisk Eggs**: In a bowl, whisk the eggs with salt and pepper.
- **Cook Omelette**: Pour eggs over the sautéed vegetables. Cook until edges set, then sprinkle cheese on top. Fold the omelette and cook until fully set.
- **Serve**: Enjoy warm.
- **Net Carbs**: Approximately 3-4 grams per serving

2. Greek Yogurt with Nuts and Berries:

Ingredients:

- 1 cup unsweetened Greek yogurt

- 1/4 cup mixed berries (blueberries, raspberries, strawberries)
- 2 tablespoons mixed nuts (almonds, walnuts)
- Optional: a drizzle of honey or a sprinkle of cinnamon

Instructions:

- **Combine Ingredients**: In a bowl, mix Greek yogurt, berries, and nuts.
- **Add Sweetener**: Drizzle with honey or sprinkle with cinnamon if desired.
- **Serve**: Enjoy as a protein-rich, satisfying breakfast.
- **Net Carbs**: Approximately 10-12 grams (depending on honey and berries)

<u>3. Quinoa Breakfast Bowl:</u>

Ingredients:

- 1/2 cup cooked quinoa
- 1/2 cup unsweetened almond milk (or milk of choice)
- 1 tablespoon chia seeds
- 1/4 cup diced apple or pear
- Cinnamon to taste
- Optional: walnuts or almonds for topping

Instructions:

- **Combine Ingredients**: In a bowl, mix quinoa, almond milk, chia seeds, and diced fruit.
- **Add Flavor**: Sprinkle with cinnamon and stir.
- **Serve**: Top with nuts if desired and enjoy warm or cold.

- **Net Carbs**: Approximately 15-17 grams (depends on fruit)

4. Avocado Toast on Whole Grain Bread:

Ingredients:

- 1 slice whole grain bread (low-carb variety)
- 1/2 ripe avocado
- Salt and pepper to taste
- Optional toppings: sliced radishes, cherry tomatoes, or a poached egg

Instructions:

- **Toast Bread**: Toast the slice of whole grain bread until golden.
- **Prepare Avocado**: Mash the avocado in a bowl and season with salt and pepper.

- **Assemble**: Spread the mashed avocado onto the toasted bread. Add optional toppings if desired.

- **Serve**: Enjoy as a satisfying breakfast.

- **Net Carbs**: Approximately 10-12 grams (depending on bread and toppings)

5. Chia Seed Pudding:

Ingredients:

- 1/4 cup chia seeds

- 1 cup unsweetened almond milk (or milk of choice)

- 1 teaspoon vanilla extract

- Optional: sweetener of choice (like stevia or honey) and fresh fruit for topping

Instructions:

- **Mix Ingredients**: In a bowl, combine chia seeds, almond milk, vanilla extract, and sweetener. Stir well.

- **Refrigerate**: Cover and refrigerate for at least 2 hours or overnight until thickened.

- **Serve**: Top with fresh fruit if desired and enjoy.

- **Net Carbs**: Approximately 10-12 grams (depends on toppings)

These breakfast recipes provide a variety of flavors and textures while supporting your maintenance phase of the Atkins Diet. Enjoy!

Phase 4: Lunch Recipes

Here are some delicious lunch recipes suitable for Phase 4 of the Atkins Diet, designed to help maintain your weight while enjoying a balanced and nutritious diet.

1. Grilled Chicken Salad:

Ingredients:

- 1 grilled chicken breast, sliced
- 2 cups mixed salad greens (spinach, arugula, romaine)
- 1/2 avocado, sliced
- 1/4 cup cherry tomatoes, halved
- 1/4 cucumber, sliced
- 2 tablespoons olive oil
- 1 tablespoon balsamic vinegar
- Salt and pepper to taste

Instructions:

- **Prepare Salad**: In a large bowl, combine salad greens, avocado, cherry tomatoes, and cucumber.

- **Add Chicken**: Top the salad with sliced grilled chicken.

- **Dress Salad**: In a small bowl, whisk together olive oil, balsamic vinegar, salt, and pepper. Drizzle over the salad.

- **Serve**: Toss gently and enjoy.

- **Net Carbs**: Approximately 8 grams per serving

2. Zucchini Noodles with Pesto and Cherry Tomatoes:

Ingredients:

- 2 medium zucchinis, spiralized
- 1 cup cherry tomatoes, halved

- 1/4 cup basil pesto (store-bought or homemade)
- 1 tablespoon olive oil
- Parmesan cheese for serving (optional)

Instructions:

- **Sauté Zoodles**: In a skillet, heat olive oil over medium heat. Add zucchini noodles and sauté for 3-4 minutes until tender.
- **Add Tomatoes**: Stir in cherry tomatoes and cook for another 1-2 minutes.
- **Toss with Pesto**: Remove from heat and toss with pesto until well coated.
- **Serve**: Top with grated Parmesan if desired and enjoy.

- **Net Carbs**: Approximately 6-8 grams per serving

3. Tuna Salad Lettuce Wraps:

Ingredients:

- 1 can (5 oz) tuna, drained
- 2 tablespoons mayonnaise
- 1 tablespoon Dijon mustard
- 1/4 cup diced celery
- Salt and pepper to taste
- Large lettuce leaves (Romaine or Butter lettuce) for wrapping

Instructions:

- **Mix Salad**: In a bowl, combine tuna, mayonnaise, Dijon mustard, diced celery, salt, and pepper.
- **Assemble Wraps**: Spoon the tuna mixture onto lettuce leaves and wrap them up.

- **Serve**: Enjoy as a refreshing, low-carb lunch.
- **Net Carbs**: Approximately 2-3 grams per wrap

4. Quinoa and Black Bean Bowl:

Ingredients:

- 1/2 cup cooked quinoa
- 1/2 cup canned black beans, rinsed and drained
- 1/4 cup corn (optional)
- 1/4 avocado, diced
- 1 tablespoon lime juice
- Chopped cilantro for garnish
- Salt and pepper to taste

Instructions:

- **Combine Ingredients**: In a bowl, mix cooked quinoa, black beans, corn, avocado, lime juice, salt, and pepper.

- **Garnish**: Top with chopped cilantro.
- **Serve**: Enjoy as a hearty, nutritious lunch.
- **Net Carbs**: Approximately 15 grams per serving (depending on corn)

5. Caprese Salad with Balsamic Reduction:

Ingredients:

- 2 large tomatoes, sliced
- 8 oz fresh mozzarella cheese, sliced
- Fresh basil leaves
- 2 tablespoons balsamic reduction
- Olive oil for drizzling
- Salt and pepper to taste

Instructions:

- **Layer Ingredients**: On a plate, alternate slices of tomato and mozzarella, adding basil leaves between layers.
- **Drizzle**: Drizzle with balsamic reduction and olive oil. Season with salt and pepper.
- **Serve**: Enjoy as a light and refreshing lunch.
- **Net Carbs**: Approximately 6 grams per serving

These lunch recipes offer a range of flavors and ingredients while supporting your maintenance phase of the Atkins Diet. Enjoy!

Phase 4: Dinner Recipes

Here are some delicious dinner recipes suitable for Phase 4 of the Atkins Diet, perfect for maintaining your weight while enjoying balanced meals.

1. Lemon Herb Grilled Shrimp with Asparagus:

Ingredients:

- 1 pound shrimp, peeled and deveined
- 2 tablespoons olive oil
- 2 tablespoons lemon juice
- 2 teaspoons dried oregano
- 1 bunch asparagus, trimmed
- Salt and pepper to taste

Instructions:

- **Marinate Shrimp**: In a bowl, combine olive oil, lemon juice, oregano, salt, and pepper. Add shrimp and marinate for 15-30 minutes.

- **Grill Asparagus**: While shrimp marinates, grill or roast asparagus until tender (about 10 minutes).

- **Grill Shrimp**: Preheat grill and cook shrimp for 2-3 minutes per side until pink and cooked through.

- **Serve**: Plate shrimp alongside asparagus and enjoy.

- **Net Carbs**: Approximately 5 grams per serving

2. Stuffed Bell Peppers:

Ingredients:

- 4 large bell peppers, halved and seeds removed
- 1 pound ground turkey or beef
- 1 cup diced tomatoes (canned, no added sugar)
- 1/2 cup cooked quinoa (optional)
- 1 teaspoon Italian seasoning
- 1/2 cup shredded cheese (optional)

Instructions:

- **Preheat Oven**: Preheat oven to 375°F (190°C).
- **Cook Filling**: In a skillet, brown ground meat. Add diced tomatoes, quinoa (if using), Italian seasoning,

salt, and pepper. Simmer for 5-10 minutes.

- **Stuff Peppers**: Fill halved bell peppers with the meat mixture. Top with cheese if desired.

- **Bake**: Place stuffed peppers in a baking dish and bake for 25-30 minutes.

- **Serve**: Enjoy warm.

- **Net Carbs**: Approximately 9 grams per stuffed pepper (depending on quinoa)

3. Zucchini Lasagna:

Ingredients:

- 2 large zucchinis, thinly sliced
- 1 pound ground beef or turkey
- 1 cup marinara sauce (low-sugar)
- 1 cup ricotta cheese
- 1 cup shredded mozzarella cheese

- 1 teaspoon Italian seasoning

- Salt and pepper to taste

Instructions:

- **Preheat Oven**: Preheat oven to 375°F (190°C).

- **Cook Meat**: In a skillet, brown ground meat. Add marinara sauce, Italian seasoning, salt, and pepper. Simmer for 5-10 minutes.

- **Layer Ingredients**: In a baking dish, layer zucchini slices, ricotta cheese, and meat sauce. Repeat layers and finish with mozzarella on top.

- **Bake**: Cover with foil and bake for 25 minutes. Remove foil and bake for another 10-15 minutes until bubbly.

- **Serve**: Let cool slightly before slicing.

- **Net Carbs**: Approximately 7 grams per serving

4. Salmon with Spinach and Feta:

Ingredients:

- 2 salmon fillets

- 2 cups fresh spinach

- 1/4 cup feta cheese, crumbled

- 2 tablespoons olive oil

- Lemon wedges for serving

- Salt and pepper to taste

Instructions:

- **Cook Spinach**: In a skillet, heat olive oil over medium heat. Add spinach and cook until wilted. Stir in feta cheese and season with salt and pepper. Set aside.

- **Cook Salmon**: In the same skillet, cook salmon fillets skin-side down for about 5-7 minutes. Flip and cook for an additional 3-4 minutes until cooked through.

- **Serve**: Plate salmon with spinach and feta on the side. Serve with lemon wedges.

- **Net Carbs**: Approximately 3 grams per serving

5. Cauliflower Fried Rice:

Ingredients:

- 1 medium head cauliflower, riced (or pre-riced cauliflower)

- 1 cup mixed vegetables (peas, carrots, bell peppers)

- 2 large eggs, beaten

- 2 tablespoons soy sauce (or tamari for gluten-free)

- 1 tablespoon sesame oil

- Green onions for garnish

Instructions:

- **Sauté Veggies**: In a large skillet, heat sesame oil over medium heat. Add mixed vegetables and sauté for 2-3 minutes.

- **Add Cauliflower**: Stir in riced cauliflower and cook for another 5-7 minutes until tender.

- **Scramble Eggs**: Push the cauliflower mixture to one side of the skillet. Add beaten eggs to the other side and scramble until cooked. Mix everything together.

- **Add Sauce**: Stir in soy sauce and garnish with green onions before serving.

- **Net Carbs**: Approximately 5 grams per serving

These dinner recipes provide variety and flavor while supporting your maintenance phase of the Atkins Diet. Enjoy!

Phase 4: Snacks Recipes

Here are some tasty snack recipes suitable for Phase 4 of the Atkins Diet, perfect for maintaining your weight while enjoying delicious treats.

1. Cucumber Slices with Hummus:

Ingredients:

- 1 cucumber, sliced
- 1/2 cup hummus (store-bought or homemade)

Instructions:

- **Slice Cucumber**: Cut cucumber into rounds.
- **Serve**: Dip cucumber slices into hummus for a refreshing snack.
- **Net Carbs**: Approximately 5-7 grams (depending on hummus)

2. Cheese Crisps:

Ingredients:

- 1 cup shredded cheese (cheddar, parmesan, or mozzarella)

Instructions:

- **Preheat Oven**: Preheat oven to 400°F (200°C).
- **Prepare Baking Sheet**: Line a baking sheet with parchment paper.

- **Form Crisps**: Place small mounds of shredded cheese on the parchment, spacing them apart. Flatten slightly.

- **Bake**: Bake for 5-7 minutes until golden and crispy. Let cool before serving.

- **Net Carbs**: Approximately 1 gram per crisp

3. Nut and Seed Trail Mix:

Ingredients:

- 1/4 cup almonds
- 1/4 cup walnuts
- 1/4 cup sunflower seeds
- Optional: a few dark chocolate chips or dried fruit (in moderation)

Instructions:

- **Mix Ingredients**: Combine nuts, seeds, and optional chocolate chips or dried fruit in a bowl.
- **Serve**: Enjoy a handful as a satisfying snack.
- **Net Carbs**: Approximately 6-8 grams per serving (depends on chocolate and dried fruit)

4. Avocado and Tuna Salad:

Ingredients:

- 1 ripe avocado, halved and pitted
- 1 can (5 oz) tuna, drained
- 1 tablespoon mayonnaise
- Salt and pepper to taste
- Lemon juice (optional)

Instructions:

- **Mix Tuna**: In a bowl, combine tuna, mayonnaise, salt, pepper, and lemon juice if desired.
- **Fill Avocado**: Spoon the tuna mixture into the avocado halves.
- **Serve**: Enjoy as a protein-rich snack.
- **Net Carbs**: Approximately 6 grams per serving

5. Egg Salad Lettuce Wraps:

Ingredients:

- 2 hard-boiled eggs, chopped
- 2 tablespoons mayonnaise
- 1 teaspoon Dijon mustard
- Salt and pepper to taste
- Large lettuce leaves for wrapping (Romaine or Butter lettuce)

Instructions:

- **Mix Salad**: In a bowl, combine chopped eggs, mayonnaise, Dijon mustard, salt, and pepper.
- **Assemble Wraps**: Spoon the egg salad onto lettuce leaves and wrap them up.
- **Serve**: Enjoy as a tasty snack.
- **Net Carbs**: Approximately 2 grams per wrap

These snack recipes offer a variety of flavors and nutrients while supporting your maintenance phase of the Atkins Diet. Enjoy!

CHAPTER SIX
Eating Out On The Atkins Diet

Eating out on the Atkins Diet can be enjoyable and easy with some planning. Here are tips and strategies to help you stay on track while dining out:

• Opt for places with customizable menus, such as steakhouses, seafood restaurants, or places that offer fresh salads. Buffets can also provide a variety of low-carb options.

• Check the restaurant's menu online before going, so you can decide on low-carb options. Look for dishes that focus on protein and non-starchy vegetables.

• Don't hesitate to request changes, like substituting fries for a side salad or vegetables. Ask for dressings and sauces on the side to control portion sizes.

• Choose grilled, baked, or roasted meats and fish. Avoid breaded or fried options. Eggs, chicken, steak, and seafood are typically great choices.

• Opt for salads with plenty of greens, cucumbers, peppers, and other low-carb veggies. Be mindful of high-carb toppings like croutons. Choose vegetable sides instead of starchy options like potatoes or rice.

• Many sauces can be high in sugars and carbs. Opt for oil and vinegar or ask about low-carb options. Avoid sugary marinades or sauces like teriyaki or barbecue.

• Drink water or unsweetened beverages. If you want something special, consider sparkling water with a twist of lemon or lime.

• Be aware that some foods may have hidden carbs (e.g., breading, sauces, or marinades). Ask questions if you're unsure about a dish's ingredients.

• If you want dessert, consider sharing with someone or opting for cheese or berries if available.

• Restaurant portions can be large. Consider sharing a meal, ordering a smaller portion, or taking leftovers home.

By keeping these tips in mind, you can enjoy dining out while staying true to your Atkins Diet goals.

Exercise And Fitness

Exercise and fitness are vital components of a healthy lifestyle, especially during weight maintenance phases like Phase 4 of the Atkins Diet. Here are some key points to consider:

- Choose exercises you genuinely enjoy to stay motivated and make fitness a regular part of your routine. This could include dancing, hiking, cycling, swimming, or group classes.

Aim for a mix of cardiovascular (aerobic) exercises, strength training, and flexibility workouts:

1. **Cardio**: Running, walking, cycling, or aerobics help improve heart health and burn calories.

2. **Strength Training**: Lifting weights or body-weight exercises (like squats and push-ups) build muscle and boost metabolism.

3. **Flexibility**: Yoga or stretching improves flexibility, balance, and relaxation.

- Establish achievable fitness goals, whether it's increasing endurance, strength, or flexibility. This helps keep you motivated and focused.

- Aim for at least 150 minutes of moderate aerobic activity or 75 minutes of vigorous activity each week, along with strength training on two or more days.

- Consistency is key for maintaining fitness and weight loss.

- Pay attention to how your body responds to different activities. Rest when needed and adjust your routine based on energy levels and recovery.

- Find opportunities to be active throughout the day. Take stairs instead of elevators, walk or bike instead of driving short distances, or incorporate short exercise breaks.

- Drink plenty of water before, during, and after exercise. Maintain a balanced diet to fuel your workouts and aid recovery.

- Consider keeping a fitness journal or using apps to track workouts, progress, and how you feel. This can help maintain motivation.

- If you're new to exercise or have specific goals, consider working with a fitness trainer or joining group classes for support and guidance.

- Allow your body time to recover with adequate rest days and sleep, as recovery is essential for progress and injury prevention.

On the Atkins Diet, you can improve your well-being, support weight maintenance, and enhance your overall health by incorporating regular physical activity into your routine.

You can maintain your weight and experience a satisfying diet by focusing on whole, nutrient-dense foods, staying hydrated, and allowing for occasional indulgences.

It is important to establish realistic fitness objectives, heed to your body, and incorporate a diverse array of exercises that you find enjoyable. These strategies will enable you to maintain your progress and maintain a healthy, balanced lifestyle. Celebrate your accomplishments and embrace the journey!

THE END